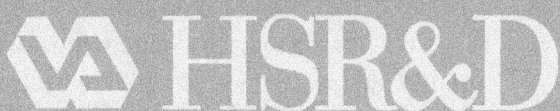

Evidence Synthesis for Determining the Efficacy of Psychotherapy for Treatment Resistant Depression

October 2009

Prepared for:

Department of Veterans Affairs
Veterans Health Administration
Health Services Research
& Development Service
Washington, DC 20420

Prepared by:

Durham Veterans Affairs Medical
Center/Duke Evidence-Based
Practice Center
Durham, NC

Investigators:

Ranak B. Trivedi, PhD
Core Investigator, Seattle VA HSR&D Center of Excellence
Research Asst. Professor, University of Washington Dept. of
Health Services, School of Public Health
Seattle, WA

Jason A. Nieuwsma, PhD
MIRECC Postdoctoral Fellow in Psychology
Durham VA Medical Center
Durham, NC

John W. Williams Jr., MD, MHS
Professor of Medicine and Psychiatry, Durham VA Medical
Center and Duke University
Director, Evidence-Based Practice Center
Durham, NC

Dana Baker, MS
Clinical Research Coordinator
Duke University
Durham, NC

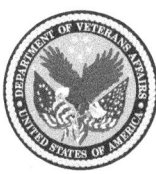

PREFACE

VA's Health Services Research and Development Service (HSR&D) works to improve the cost, quality, and outcomes of health care for our nation's veterans. Collaborating with VA leaders, managers, and policy makers, HSR&D focuses on important health care topics that are likely to have significant impact on quality improvement efforts. One significant collaborative effort is HSR&D's Evidence-based Synthesis Program (ESP). Through this program, HSR&D provides timely and accurate evidence syntheses on targeted health care topics. These products will be disseminated broadly throughout VA and will: inform VA clinical policy, develop clinical practice guidelines, set directions for future research to address gaps in knowledge, identify the evidence to support VA performance measures, and rationalize drug formulary decisions.

HSR&D provided funding for the two Evidence Based Practice Centers (EPCs) supported by the Agency for Healthcare Research and Quality (AHRQ) that also had an active and publicly acknowledged VA affiliation—Southern California EPC and Portland, OR EPC—so they could develop evidence syntheses on requested topics for dissemination to VA policymakers. A planning committee with representation from HSR&D, Patient Care Services, Office of Quality and Performance, and the VISN Clinical Management Officers, has been established to identify priority topics and to ensure the quality of final reports. Comments on this evidence report are welcome and can be sent to Susan Schiffner, ESP Program Manager, at Susan.Schiffner@va.gov.

TABLE OF CONTENTS

TABLES

FIGURES

EXECUTIVE SUMMARY

BACKGROUND

Major depressive disorder (MDD) is a prevalent disorder impacting an estimated 13% of the general population, and a third of the veteran population. Of the patients who experience at least one depressive episode, approximately 20% will experience chronic depression and 60-85% will experience recurrence and relapse. Antidepressant medications are the most commonly prescribed treatment modality for MDD and are often the first line of treatment in primary care settings. However, fewer than 50% of patients fully remit after adequate dosage of antidepressant treatment. Treatment options for these "treatment resistant" patients vary but typically involve using other psychoactive medications as augmentation (i.e., addition of another medication) or substitution treatment (i.e., switching medications). Less attention has been paid to using psychotherapy as an augmentation or substitution treatment for treatment resistant patients, despite psychotherapy being associated with clinical improvements in MDD comparable to those achieved with antidepressants. The current review will address the effectiveness of psychotherapeutic approaches as a second step treatment for MDD in patients who do not achieve remission after initial treatment with antidepressants.

Question: In primary care patients with major depressive disorder who do not achieve remission with acute phase antidepressant treatment, is empirically based psychotherapy used as an augmentation or substitution treatment more effective than control for achieving remission?

METHODS

We searched PubMed from 1950-2009 using standard search terms. Titles, abstracts, and articles were reviewed in duplicate. Extant literature was initially screened for relevant systematic reviews. Following this, primary literature was screened for relevant randomized clinical trials comparing medications to psychotherapy in patients with major depressive disorder. Data were extracted in duplicate in articles that were included in this review. We evaluated study quality for the primary literature. All data were summarized in evidence tables and in narrative.

RESULTS

We initially screened 41 systematic reviews, of which 29 were excluded at the title/abstract level and the remaining 12 were excluded after full-text review. For the primary literature, 333 titles were screened, of which 290 were excluded at the title/abstract level and 31 were excluded after full-text review. The remaining 12 articles reflected five unique randomized clinical trials examining the effect of psychotherapy in patients who had shown resistance to antidepressant therapy. Because one of the trials had both "substitution with psychotherapy" and "augmentation with psychotherapy" arms, these were treated as two different studies, resulting in a total of six studies reviewed. A total of 567 patients were evaluated; none of these were recruited from VA clinics. Psychotherapy was examined as an augmentation to antidepressant medication in four studies and as a substitution treatment to replace medication in two studies. The STAR*D trial examined psychotherapy in both conditions. Three studies-including the two STAR*D treatment arms- were rated as good quality, two studies were rated fair, and one was rated poor. The STAR*D trial used an equipoise stratified randomization design; the remaining four studies were true RCTs. Patients in the comparison groups were on medications in all studies.

A fair quality trial compared psychotherapy as augmentation treatment to medication by randomizing 24 patients to either a 16-session dialectical behavior therapy (DBT) group or to a wait list condition. Participants in the DBT group evidenced significantly more improvement than participants in the wait list condition, both on interviewer rated and self-report measures of depression severity. Interpretation is complicated by control participants being allowed to continue in individual therapy.

Psychotherapy was also examined as an augmentation treatment to medication in a fair quality trial, in which 44 patients were randomized to either 12 sessions of cognitive therapy or to lithium augmentation. Participants in the lithium augmentation condition evidenced significantly more improvement than participants in the cognitive therapy condition on an interviewer rated measure of depression severity, but there were no between-group differences on a self-report measure of depression severity. One limitation was that patients must have partially responded to medication treatment to be eligible for inclusion.

A moderate sized, good quality trial also used psychotherapy to augment antidepressant treatment. In this study, 158 patients were randomized to either 16 sessions of cognitive therapy (CT) or to clinical management with antidepressant medication. Participants in both conditions improved over time but there were no significant differences between the two treatment groups.

The good quality STAR*D trial examined psychotherapy and medication as either augmentation or substitution treatments to initial treatment with citalopram. Sixteen sessions of CT were provided, although only a minority of enrolled participants completed all sessions. Only the portion of results germane to our question was considered for the review, resulting in a sample size of 304 participants. Patients were allowed to refuse randomization to treatment strategies that they found unacceptable, resulting in the two CT conditions having roughly half the number of participants as in the two medication conditions. While participants in all four conditions evidenced improvement over time, there were no significant differences between the conditions. However, participants who had citalopram augmented with another antidepressant did demonstrate quicker benefit than participants who had citalopram augmented with cognitive therapy. This study had excellent ecological validity given that patient preferences were taken into account prior to randomization.

Finally, a poor quality study by Blackburn and Moore (1997), examined psychotherapy as a substitution treatment to replace antidepressant medication. There were 37 patients in this study who were randomized to 27 sessions of psychotherapy over two years or to clinical management with antidepressant medication. While participants in both conditions evidenced clinical improvement over time, there were no significant differences between the two conditions.

SUMMARY

In summary, two good quality, moderate-sized trials showed equal benefit from augmenting antidepressant medication with CT and from active medication management, one fair quality small study showed lithium augmentation to be more beneficial than CT, and one fair quality trial showed short-term benefit from augmentation through 16 sessions of DBT. A moderate-sized, good quality study and a small, poor quality study found equal benefit from substituting CT for antidepressant treatment and from continuing management of depression with medication. There was significant heterogeneity in study designs, sample sizes, and comparator groups, and most studies were underpowered to detect moderate effect sizes. We conclude that current trials do not support favoring psychotherapy over antidepressant medication for mid-life adults with treatment resistant MDD; however, psychotherapy appears to be an equally effective treatment compared to antidepressant medication and is therefore a reasonable treatment option for this demographic. Whether these results are directly applicable to Veterans is uncertain because most study samples were mid-life adults, more than 50% female, and medical and psychiatric co-morbidity was incompletely described. The limited number of studies, mixed effects and uncertain applicability to Veterans suggest a need for additional trials to adequately evaluate the potential treatment benefit of psychotherapy for treatment resistant depression.

EVIDENCE REPORT

INTRODUCTION

Major depressive disorder (MDD) is one of the leading causes of disability worldwide. 1 The lifetime prevalence of MDD in the general population is estimated at 13%[2], of which approximately 20% will experience chronic depression and 60-85% will experience recurrence and relapse.[3] This number is even higher in the VA medical system, where an estimated one third of veterans experience MDD.[4] MDD is associated with greater health care utilization, greater functional impairment, and increased mortality.[2] In addition, subclinical symptoms of depression can reduce quality of life, worsen disability, and adversely affect co-existing chronic medical conditions.[5-8] Both antidepressant medications and depression-specific psychotherapies are effective as first-line treatments for MDD. In primary care settings, most patients with MDD are treated with antidepressant medications, but a substantial proportion of patients fail to recover with this initial treatment. This evidence synthesis was requested to evaluate the efficacy of psychological treatments as step-2 treatment for patients with MDD who do not achieve remission with an initial course of antidepressant medication.

BACKGROUND

Antidepressant medications are the most commonly prescribed treatment modality in MDD.[9] The most recent American Psychiatric Association (APA) guidelines[10] suggest the use of antidepressants for mild, moderate or severe depressive disorders, a position that has remained consistent in the more recent "guideline watch" by Fochtmann & Gelenberg (2008).[11] The efficacy and effectiveness of antidepressant treatment in primary care have been demonstrated in multiple large scale studies and systematic reviews.[12-16] Several classes and types of antidepressants exist which do not substantially differ in their efficacy or effectiveness for treating MDD.[17] Therefore, primary care physicians have a wide array of antidepressant options that they may prescribe depending on suitability to patient, patient preference, affordability, side effect profile, and the targeted physiological system.[17]

In addition, a sizeable body of literature has examined the efficacy and effectiveness of psychotherapy as acute phase treatment for MDD, either as monotherapy or in combination with antidepressant treatment. Psychotherapy is a heterogeneous class of treatments in which the therapist utilizes interpersonal strategies with the intention of alleviating mental or emotion distress.[18] Cognitive therapy (CT) is the most widely studied form of psychotherapy for depression, although many other psychotherapeutic modalities exist that are depression-specific, empirically validated, and accessible through referral or adoption by the primary care team. Recent reviews and meta-analyses of acute phase treatment for depression have shown that psychotherapy may be as effective as antidepressant treatment and more effective than usual care in treating mild, moderate, and severe MDD.[19-23] When MDD is severe, chronic or recurrent, the combination of medication and psychotherapy as initial treatment appears to be indicated.[17] Combination of psychotherapy with an antidepressant has demonstrated greater treatment gains, lower relapse rates, and increased adherence to treatment when compared to usual care or antidepressant monotherapy.[24-27] Therefore, current evidence suggests that antidepressants and psychotherapy may both form effective first line treatments in patients with MDD, individually or in combination.

However, response to initial treatment for MDD remains poor even when treatment recommendations are rigorously followed.[28, 29] Fewer than 50% of patients fully remit after an adequate trial of antidepressant medication or psychotherapy.[30, 31] Patients who do not fully remit are often considered "treatment resistant" or "treatment refractory." Treatment resistant depression (TRD) is typically defined as an inadequate response to at least one 6-week or longer trial of an antidepressant at an adequate dose.[32] TRD does not include patients who did not adhere to initial treatment recommendations. Clinical factors associated with treatment resistant depression (TRD) include comorbid generalized anxiety and other Axis I disorders (e.g., phobias), early onset of MDD, previous suicide attempts, number of prior depressive episodes, older age, and unemployment.[33-36] In primary care settings, these findings may help physicians *a priori* determine patients who may be most at-risk for TRD.

Primary care physicians have several options when treating patients with TRD: augmenting treatment by adding another medication; switching to a different antidepressant; augmenting treatment through adding psychotherapy; and switching from medication to psychotherapy.[37] However, studies of clinical practice suggest that medications are often the only active treatment provided by primary care providers as a second step treatment for MDD.[17, 38] Several limitations to this approach should be noted. First, the addition of another antidepressant may increase the number and/or severity of side effects that patients experience. Side effects are known to reduce quality of life and increase the chances of non-adherence, interfering with the treatment of MDD.[39] Second, focus on antidepressants may ignore the potential impact of psychosocial factors in TRD. For instance, cognitions and behaviors related to MDD may be interfering with the treatment regimen and may best be modified by skills training. This is especially true when patients are experiencing acute stressors (e.g., bereavement), where psychotherapy may improve patients' long-term outcomes.[23] Third, patients may simply not respond to antidepressant treatment or may not prefer taking medications. In all of these scenarios, the addition or substitution of psychotherapy may be a preferred alternative.

In summary, psychotherapy and pharmacotherapy appear to be equally effective as initial approaches to treating MDD in primary care. However, approximately half of patients do not remit after initial treatment even when treatment regimens are rigorously followed. Switching to a different antidepressant or augmenting treatment by adding a second antidepressant medication are both common clinical practices that are recommended in current guidelines as second step treatment strategies. However, the addition or substitution of psychotherapy is not addressed as a step-2 treatment for MDD in published guidelines.

Therefore, the focus of the current review is two-fold:
To review literature examining the use of psychotherapy as a second line treatment for patients with depression who do not remit with initial antidepressant medication; and,
To determine the applicability of these studies to VA patients treated in primary care settings.

The purpose of this review was to generate guidelines that would help determine whether the use of psychotherapy, either as an augmentation or a switch strategy, would lead to better outcomes in patients who had not responded to initial adequate antidepressant treatment.

METHODS

TOPIC DEVELOPMENT

The Veterans Health Administration (VHA) uses quality improvement strategies, including clinical practice guidelines, clinical reminders in the electronic medical record, and performance measurement to improve care processes. For veterans with depression and other mental illnesses managed in primary care settings, the VHA has recently made major investments in integrated primary care-mental health programs. This project was nominated by Ira Katz, Deputy Chief, Patient Care Services for Mental Health, and Carla Cassidy and Joe Francis, Office of Quality and Performance, with input from a technical expert panel. The overall goal was to synthesize data on the efficacy of psychotherapy in patients who do not fully remit with adequate antidepressant treatment.

Therefore, the key question was as follows:
In primary care patients with major depressive disorder who do not achieve remission with acute phase antidepressant treatment, is empirically based psychotherapy used as an augmentation or substitution treatment more effective than control for achieving remission?

For the purposes of this review, cognitive therapy (CT), interpersonal therapy (IPT), problem-solving therapy, dialectical behavior therapy (DBT), acceptance and commitment therapy (ACT), and mindfulness based cognitive therapy (MBCT) were considered as empirically based psychotherapies.

SEARCH STRATEGY

We searched PubMed between 1950 and February 26, 2009 using standard search terms. Appendix A provides details of the search terms. Our strategy was twofold. First, we attempted to identify a good quality, relevant systematic review that would summarize the extant literature. If identified, our strategy would be to search for randomized clinical trials since the original review. No such systematic review was identified. Consequently, we searched PubMed for relevant randomized clinical trials (RCT). Titles, abstracts and full text articles were reviewed in duplicate. Data were extracted in duplicate from articles meeting all inclusion criteria. We then rated the overall quality of each study, assigned a grade, and summarized the data in narrative. Eligible articles were imported into an electronic reference database (EndNote® XI).

STUDY SELECTION

Two trained researchers independently reviewed the titles and/or abstracts of citations identified through the PubMed literature search. If articles did not clearly meet the inclusion criteria, they were excluded at the title and abstract level. The remaining articles were identified for full text review, at which stage those that did not meet inclusion criteria were excluded. In case of disagreement, the two reviewers met to identify and resolve the disagreement. To be eligible, the articles had to be published in English, and include:

- English-speaking adult outpatients from general medical settings.
- Randomized clinical trial involving at least one of the following psychotherapy modalities: cognitive behavior therapy (CBT), interpersonal therapy (IPT), problem-solving therapy, dialectical behavior therapy (DBT), acceptance and commitment therapy (ACT), or mindfulness based cognitive therapy (MBCT).
- Patients with resistant MDD, defined as a sample consisting of at least 80% with either no remission or partial remission after being treated with adequate dose of an antidepressant for at least six weeks.
- Articles were excluded if patients were receiving psychotherapy at the time of recruitment, and/or if patients had comorbid psychiatric conditions that required specialty psychiatric care. These included, but were not limited to, active suicidal or parasuicidal ideation, severe substance abuse, or borderline personality disorder.

DATA ABSTRACTION

The following data were abstracted on the included studies: definition of persistence; type of psychotherapy; type of comparison group; setting (primary care/mental health clinic); VA (Yes/No); sample size; study-specific inclusion/exclusion criteria; age/sex/race of sample; indices of MDD severity (duration of current episode; number of prior episodes; number of hospitalizations; number of suicide attempts); data on interviewer-rated depression severity (if applicable); data on self-reported depression severity (if applicable); duration of follow-up. All data were abstracted by one reviewer with oversight being provided by the other reviewer. All disagreements were resolved using discussion and consensus.

QUALITY ASSESSMENT

Quality of selected articles was assessed using the quality rating tool described in Appendix C. We abstracted data on completeness of follow-up (<30% drop-out rate, <10% differential drop-out rate); method to address incomplete data; adequacy of randomization; adequacy of allocation concealment; outcome assessment blind to intervention allocation; and whether there was a conflict of interest, either stated or implied.

DATA SYNTHESIS

We constructed evidence tables showing the study characteristics and results for all included articles, organized by the unique studies from which they were derived. We critically analyzed studies to compare characteristics, methods, and findings. We compiled a summary of findings and drew conclusions based on qualitative synthesis of the findings.

PEER REVIEW

A draft version of this report was sent to three peer reviewers. Their comments and our responses are presented in Appendix B.

RESULTS

LITERATURE FLOW

Using the search strategy described in Appendix A, 41 systematic reviews were identified, of which 29 were excluded at the title and abstract level and the remaining 12 were excluded after conducting a full-text review (Figure 1). Reviews were excluded primarily because they did not apply to the question we were addressing or were not systematic; therefore, no systematic reviews were included in this report.

Next, we searched for relevant randomized clinical trials. Using the search strategy described in Appendix B, 333 randomized clinical trials were identified for review. Of these, 290 were excluded at the title and abstract level, and 43 were selected for full text review. Thirty-one articles were excluded following full-text review, yielding 12 articles for inclusion (Figure 2). These 12 articles represent five unique studies, of which one of the studies (STAR*D trial) used both augmentation and substitution treatment modalities in separate treatment arms, each with a unique comparison group. These two arms were treated as separate studies in this review. Therefore, the evidence tables and narrative summarize six studies, with the caveat that two of the studies represented separate arms of the same trial. Full consensus was achieved between the two reviewers at each stage.

SAMPLE CHARACTERISTICS

A total of 567 patients were evaluated across the studies. Patients were recruited from both mental health clinics (MHC) and primary care (PC) clinics. Three studies were conducted in the United States, two in Great Britain, and one in Canada. None of the studies recruited participants from VA clinics. Sample sizes ranged from 24 to 304 participants; two studies contributed 81% of the subjects.[37, 40] Across all studies, participants' average age was approximately 40-years-old, females compromised half to three quarters of the studies' participants, and Caucasians represented at least 75% of the racial makeup in studies that reported ethnicity. The average length of patients' current depressive episodes ranged from 30 to 123 weeks, with the average number of lifetime depressive episodes ranging from 2.2 to 8.5. For all studies, depression severity was moderate as determined by self-report measures. These characteristics are summarized in Table 1 and show significant heterogeneity in depression severity and chronicity. Sample characteristics for the psychotherapy and the comparison groups are provided if reported.

Table 1: Sample Characteristics

Study	Harley et al., 2008	Kennedy et al., 2003	Scott et al., 2000	Thase et al., 2007 (Augmentation Arm)	Thase et al., 2007 (Substitution Arm)	Blackburn & Moore, 1997*[†]
Sample size, n						
Psychotherapy	13	23	80	65	36	17
Comparator	11	21	78	117	86	20
Age, y (M±SD)						
Psychotherapy		40.7±12.5	43.5 ± 9.8	40.6 ± 11.5	43.4 ± 14.7	37.8 ± 13.1
Comparator	41.8	37.7±11.3	43.2 ±11.2	39.7 ± 13.5	41.5 ± 13.3	40.1 ± 12.7
Female, n						
Psychotherapy		12 (52%)	37 (46%)	41 (63%)	22 (61%)	17 (77%)*
Comparator	18 (75%)	12 (57%)	41 (53%)	78 (67%)	53 (62%)	17 (65%)*
Caucasian, n		–	–			–
Psychotherapy				52 (80%)	28 (78%)	
Comparator	20 (83%)			99 (85%)	63 (73%)	
Duration of current episode, wks (M±SD)						
Psychotherapy	28.7 ± 18.8	126 ± 170	62.9	129 ± 214	76 ± 135	30.4 ± 6.1
Comparator	41.8 ± 53.6	120 ± 161	56.4	87 ± 206	115 ± 234	29.9 ± 5.6
Number of prior MDD episodes (M±SD)						
Psychotherapy	Not	2.1± 1.5	2 (median)	7.3 ± 14.1	8.7 ± 18.8	4.1 ± 3.4
Comparator	Reported	2.3 ± 1.4	2 (median)	4.6 ± 5.4	8.4 ± 16.0	3.2 ± 2.2
Baseline HAM-D[a] scores						
Psychotherapy	16.2 ± 4.5	12.1 ± 2.2	12.1 ± 2.7	17.8 ± 5.7	16.4 ± 6.2	11.8 ± 6.3
Comparator	18.6 ± 4.7	11.6 ± 1.9	12.2 ± 2.9	16.0 ± 6.7	16.0 ± 6.7	10.6 ± 6.8
Baseline self-report scores	BDI[b]	BDI	BDI	QIDS-SR[c]	QIDS-SR	BDI
Psychotherapy	27.3 ± 8.8	22.7 ± 8.6	21.7 ± 7.7	11.9 ± 4.3	11.2 ± 4.3	20.4 ± 11.1
Comparator	27.4 ± 11.7	22.4 ± 10.3	22.3 ± 8.0	12.0 ± 4.6	12.1 ± 4.6	19.7 ± 14.2
Setting	MHC[d]	MHC	MHC	MHC & PC[e]	MHC & PC	MHC
Location	Boston, MA	Canada	England	U.S.A.	U.S.A.	Scotland

*[†]HAM-D, BDI and QIDS-SR scores based on smaller number that enrolled in phase 2 of the study following initial treatment with ADM

[a] HAM-D=Hamiltion Depresion Scale; [b]BDI=Beck Depression Inventory; [bc]QIDS-SR=Quick Inventory of Depressive Symptoms-Self Report; [d]MHC=Mental Health Clinic; [e]PC=Primary Care Clinic

To determine persistence, studies used different criteria but followed similar methodology. First, authors ensured that patients had a MDD at baseline. Second, patients underwent antidepressant (AD) treatment at adequate dose as first step treatment. Third, authors ensured that patients continued to have residual symptoms of MDD. All studies except Harley et al. (2008) reported criteria used to determine initial depression diagnosis. Two studies provided 1st step AD treatment whereas the others relied on non-study practitioners. HAM-D scores, either singly or in combination with BDI scores, were used predominantly to determine residual depression following AD treatment. The various criteria used to determine persistence are summarized in Table 2.

Table 2: Criteria to Determine Persistent Depression

Study	Harley et al., 2008	Kennedy et al., 2003	Scott et al., 2000	Thase et al., 2007	Blackburn & Moore, 1997
Criteria for initial depression diagnosis	Not Reported	HAM-D=17≥16	MDD episode in previous 18 months according to DSM-III-R; residual symptoms for ≥8 weeks	Hx of MDD; HAM-D≥14	Unipolar MDD using SADS[a]; HAM-D≥16
1st step AD[b] treatment: Type and Dosage	As prescribed by non-study psychiatrists	Moclobemide (300-600 mg/day) OR Paroxetine (20-40 mg/day) OR Sertraline (50-200 mg/day) OR Venlafaxine (75-225 mg/day)	Tricyclic antidepressant, SSRI, atypical AD, or MAOI; Minimum dose equivalent to 125 mg of amitriptyline)	Citalopram 20 mg/day titrated to 40 mg by week 4 if needed; Max. 60 mg/day by week 6	As prescribed by non-study practitioners; Equivalent to 100 mg amitryptiline OR 45 mg phenelzine OR 20 mg of Sertraline
1st Step AD Treatment: Duration	≥6 weeks	8-14 weeks	≥8 weeks (at least 4 weeks of adequate dose)	14 weeks	16 weeks
Was 1st AD step treatment provided in the study?	No	Yes	No	Yes	No
Criteria to Determine Persistence Following 1st Step AD Treatment	MDD on SCID-I[c]	HAM-D=8-15	HAM-D≥8 & BDI≥9	HAM-D≥14	Moderate symptoms on BDI and HAM-D>11

[a]SADS=Schedule for Affective Disorders and Schizophrenia; [b]AD=Antidepressant; [c]SCID-I=Structured Clinical Interview for DSM-III-R, I

STUDY DESIGN & INTERVENTIONS

Four studies used true randomization whereas the two studies from the STAR*D trial used an equipoise stratified randomization design, allowing patients to refuse to be randomized to treatments that would not be acceptable. Follow-up durations ranged from 8 to 104 weeks. Psychotherapy was examined as an augmentation treatment with antidepressant medication in four studies and as a substitution treatment replacing medication in two studies. In terms of the modality of psychotherapy provided, one small study used DBT41 whereas all others used CT.

All patients in the comparison groups were taking antidepressant medications, from a wide array of antidepressant classes. Three of the comparison groups received medication in a maintenance wait list condition, and three of the comparison groups received an active systematic alteration to their medication regimens (including both arms of the STAR*D trial). Retention rates in the different conditions ranged from 25% to 91%.

All studies used the Hamilton Depression Rating Scale (HAM-D) as their clinician administered diagnostic tool. Four studies used the Beck Depression Inventory (BDI) as their self-report measure whereas the two STAR*D trial studies used the QIDS-SR as their self-report measure. Mean baseline scores ranged from 11.2 to 17.3 on the HAM-D and from 20.0 to 27.3 on the BDI. Three trials were identified as good quality studies, two studies as fair, and one study as poor. Only three studies reported a sample size calculation. Study design and intervention overview is provided in Table 3.

Table 3: Study Design and Interventions

Study	Harley et al., 2008	Kennedy et al., 2003	Scott et al., 2000	Thase et al., 2007 (Augment)	Thase et al., 2007 (Substitute)	Blackburn & Moore, 1997
Duration of follow up, wks	16	8	20	14	14	104
Study design	RCT	RCT	RCT	Equipoise Stratified RCT	Equipoise Stratified RCT	RCT
Augmentation with Medication, or Substitution?	Augment	Augment	Augment	Augment	Substitute	Substitute
Psychotherapy Intervention Used	DBT[a] Group	CT[b]	CT	CT	CT	CT
# of sessions	16	12	16	24	24	27
Comparator	ADM[c] Continue	Lithium Augment	ADM Continue	ADM Augment	ADM Switch	ADM Continue
Power calculation	No	No	Yes	Yes	Yes	No
Quality rating	Fair	Fair	Good	Good	Good	Poor

[a]DBT=Dialectical Behavior Therapy; [b]CT=Cognitive Therapy; [c]ADM=Antidepressant Medication; [d]NS=Not Significant

STUDY RESULTS

Results from the six studies are summarized in Table 4 and are described in detail next. The four studies that describe psychotherapy as augmentation treatment are described first, followed by the two studies that used psychotherapy as a substitute for medications.

Psychotherapy as Augmentation to Antidepressant Medication

Harley et al. (2008) examined psychotherapy as an augmentation treatment to medication by randomizing 24 patients to either a DBT group (n=13) or to a wait list condition (WL; n=11).[41] Patients in the DBT condition received 16 weekly sessions of a 90-minute coping skills group in addition to remaining on antidepressant medication, while patients in the WL condition continued taking antidepressant medication and meeting with their psychiatrists and healthcare providers as usual. Treatment resistance in this study was defined as current depression determined by a structured evaluation after stable, adequate treatment with antidepressant medication for at least six weeks. Post treatment analyses found significant differences between the two groups for mean scores on the HAM-D (DBT=11.3; WL=17.1; F = 4.63, $p < .05$) and BDI (DBT=15.1; WL=25.9; F = 9.50, $p < .01$), such that patients in the DBT group evidenced more clinical improvement than those in the WL condition. The retention rate was 77% in the DBT group and 82% in the WL condition. Given the small sample size and confound of allowing patients to continue in non-CBT individual therapy, we assigned an overall quality rating of "fair" to this study.

Kennedy et al. (2003) examined psychotherapy as an augmentation treatment to medication by randomizing 44 patients to either cognitive therapy (CT; n=23) or lithium augmentation (LA; n=21).[42] Patients in the CT condition received 12 psychotherapy sessions delivered over eight weeks and were seen every four weeks for a medication checkup, while patients in the LA condition had their antidepressant medication augmented with lithium carbonate (starting dose of 600mg/day) and were seen every two weeks for clinical management. Treatment resistance in this study was defined as having a HAM-D score between 8 and 15 after 8-14 weeks of treatment with antidepressant medication. Post treatment analyses found a significant difference between the two groups for mean scores on the HAM-D (CT=14.8; LA=9.2; t = 2.02, $p = .04$), such that patients in the LA condition showed a greater decrease in depressive symptoms than those in the CT condition. No significant post treatment difference was found between the two groups for mean scores on the BDI (CT=19.9; LA=15.1). The retention rate was 74% in the CT condition and 71% in the LA condition. One limitation of this study is that it only included "partial responders" to initial antidepressant medication treatment (i.e., HAM-D score from 8 to 15) and excluded "non-responders" (i.e., HAM-D $\geq$ 16). It also did not report a sample size calculation and probably lacked sufficient statistical power to detect clinically important differences. We assigned an overall quality rating of "fair" to this study.

Multiple articles were identified for a study that examined psychotherapy as an augmentation treatment to medication.[40, 43-46] Data were primarily extracted from Scott et al. (2000).[40] In this good quality study, 158 patients were randomized to either CT (n=80) or clinical management (CM; n=78). An analysis of the pre-set sample size of 160 gave 80% power to detect a reduction in relapse rates from 40% in one group to 20% in the other at $p = .05$. Patients in the CT condition received 16 psychotherapy sessions over 20 weeks in addition to continuing on antidepressant medication, while patients in the CM condition continued on antidepressant treatment and were seen every four weeks for 30-minite medication management appointments. Treatment resistance in this study was defined as having a HAM-D score ≥ 8 and BDI score ≥ 9 after at least eight weeks of adequate treatment with an antidepressant medication. Participants had an average age of 43 and 49% were female. The average duration of participants' current depressive episode was 60 weeks (CT=63; CM=56), with both groups having a median of two lifetime episodes of depression. While participants in both conditions improved, post treatment analyses found no significant differences between the two groups for mean scores on the HAM-D (CT=8.7; CM=9.4) or BDI (CT=13.8; CM=16.1). Retention was measured as staying in until relapse or until the end of the study at 68 weeks, resulting in a 76% retention rate in the CT condition and an 85% retention rate in the CM condition. A limitation of this study is that it allowed for patients with partially remitted depressive symptoms and no diagnosis of current major depression to participate.

The STAR*D trial[32, 37, 47, 48] was a multistage, multicenter trial that examined both psychotherapy and medication as either augmentation or substitution treatments to initial treatment with citalopram. Treatment resistance in the STAR*D trial was defined as having a HAM-D score ≥ 14 after 14 weeks of treatment with citalopram. The equipoise-stratified randomization design employed in this study allowed patients to refuse randomization to treatment strategies that they found unacceptable, which resulted in asymmetrical sample sizes for different treatment arms. Less than one third of participants agreed to true randomization, which is a significant limitation of the study in terms of internal validity. Analyses conducted prior to data collection indicate that too few patients were randomized to the different treatment conditions to achieve the originally desired power. However, this study represents the best external validity given that they accounted for patient preferences, which is similar to what may be expected in primary care settings. We assigned an overall quality rating of "good" to both the augmentation and substitution arms of this study. Data are presented separately below, first examining psychotherapy and medication as an augmentation to citalopram and then examining psychotherapy and medication as substitution treatments to replace citalopram. Data were primarily extracted from Thase et al. (2007).[37]

In the augmentation arm, 182 patients were assigned to either augmentation cognitive therapy (A-CT; n=65) or augmentation antidepressant medication (A-ADM; n=117). Patients in the A-CT condition received 16 psychotherapy sessions over 12 weeks in addition to continuing on citalopram, while patients in the A-ADM condition had their treatment with citalopram augmented with either bupropion or buspirone. Participants had an average age of 40, 65% were female, and 83% were Caucasian. The average duration of participants' current depressive episode was 102 weeks (A-CT=129; A-ADM=87), with a mean of 5.6 lifetime episodes of depression (A-CT=7.3; A-ADM=4.6). There were no significant between-group differences in mean baseline depression scores on the HAM-D (A-CT=17.8; A-ADM=16.0) or QIDS-C (A-CT=11.9; A-ADM=12.0). While participants in both conditions evidenced significant improvement, post treatment analyses found no significant differences between the two groups for percent remitted on the HAM-D (A-CT=23.1%; A-ADM=33.3%) or for mean scores on the QIDS-C (A-CT=8.2; A-ADM=8.2). However, participants in the A-ADM condition did demonstrate quicker benefit than participants in the A-CT condition. The retention rate was 91% in the A-CT condition (although only 27% of patients completed at least 16 sessions) and 81% in the A-ADM condition.

In summary, the two good quality, moderate sized trials showed equal benefit from augmenting antidepressant medication with 16 to 24 sessions of cognitive therapy and from active management of depression with medication, whereas a small fair quality study showed greater benefit from lithium augmentation than cognitive therapy augmentation. A single fair quality trial showed short-term benefit from 16 sessions of DBT. Because study populations and designs were conceptually heterogeneous, a summary estimate of effect was not calculated.

Psychotherapy as Step-2 Substitution for Antidepressant Medication

In the substitution arm of STAR*D, 122 patients were randomized using an equipoise-stratified randomization design to either substitution cognitive therapy (S-CT; n=36) or substitution antidepressant medication (S-ADM; n=86). Patients in the S-CT condition discontinued treatment with citalopram and received 16 psychotherapy sessions over 12 weeks, while patients in the S-ADM condition discontinued citalopram and switched to treatment with bupropion, sertraline, or venlafaxine. Participants had an average age of 42, 61% were female, and 75% were Caucasian. The average duration of participants' current depressive episode was 103 weeks (S-CT=76; S-ADM=115), with a mean of 8.5 lifetime episodes of depression (S-CT=8.7; S-ADM=8.4). There were no significant between-group differences in mean baseline depression scores on the HAM-D (S-CT=16.4; S-ADM=16.0) or QID-S (S-CT=11.2; S-ADM=12.1). While participants in both conditions evidenced significant improvement, post treatment analyses found no significant differences between the two groups for percent remitted on the HAM-D (S-CT=25.0%; S-ADM=27.9%) or for mean scores on the QID-S (S-CT=9.1; S-ADM=9.1). The retention rate was 83% in the S-CT condition (although only 35% completed at least 16 sessions) and 73% in the S-ADM condition.

The poor quality study by Blackburn and Moore (1997) examined psychotherapy as a substitution treatment to replace antidepressant medication by randomizing 37 patients to either CT (n=17) or antidepressant medication (ADM; n=20).[49] Patients in the CT condition received 27 psychotherapy sessions over 104 weeks, while patients in the ADM condition continued on an antidepressant medication of their prescriber's choice (prescribers were also free to switch medications) and were seen by their providers about every three weeks. Treatment resistance was not specifically defined in this study, but after 16 weeks of treatment with an antidepressant medication, patients continued to have depressive symptoms at a level comparable to that of the other patient populations included in this review (see Table 1). Post treatment analyses found no significant differences between the two groups for mean scores on the HAM-D (CT=8.6; ADM=9.3) or BDI (CT=14.2; ADM=18.1). The retention rate was 35% in the CT condition and was 25% in the ADM condition. The "poor" quality rating was based on the poor retention rate, lack of statistical power, unorthodox length of CT treatment protocol, and lack of operational definition for treatment resistance.

In summary, a moderate-sized, good quality study and a small, poor quality study found equal benefit from substituting cognitive therapy for antidepressant treatment and from continuing management of depression with medication in patients with treatment resistant MDD.

Table 4: Results of the Psychotherapy Intervention

Study	Harley et al., 2008	Kennedy et al., 2003	Scott et al., 2000	Thase et al., 2007 (Aug-mentation)	Thase et al., 2007 (Substitution)	Blackburn & Moore, 1997
Retention rate, n *Psychotherapy* *Comparator*	10 (77%) 9 (82%)	17 (74%) 15 (71%)	61 (76%) 66 (85%)	59 (91%) 95 (81%)	30 (83%) 63 (73%)	6 (35%) 5 (25%)
Post-treatment HAM-D Scores (M±SD) *Psychotherapy* *Comparator* *Effect Size*	11.3 ± 5.3 17.1 ± 6.2 d=1.45	14.8 ± 9.9 9.2 ± 6.7 d=.32	8.7±5.3 9.4 ± 5.3 NS[a]	Remission: 23.1% 33.3% NS	Remission: 25.0% 27.9% NS	8.6±5.6 9.3±7.2 NS
Post-treatment BDI Scores (M±SD) *Psychotherapy* *Comparator* *Effect Size*	15.1 ±12.1 25.9±16.3 d=1.31	19.9 ± 10.3 15.1 ±11.4 NS	13.8 ±9.6 16.1 ± 10.0 NS	8.2 ±5.1 8.2 ± 4.8 NS*	9.1 ± 5.4 9.1 ± 5.0 NS*	14.2 ± 9.9 18.1 ± 13.1 NS
Quality rating	Fair	Fair	Good	Good	Good	Poor

[a] NS=Not significant at p<.05; *Results are for QIDS-C

SUMMARY AND DISCUSSION

The key observation that emerges from review of the literature is that current evidence examining the effect of psychotherapy as augmentation or substitute therapy in resistant depression is sparse and reveals mixed results. Of the six studies reviewed, four studies examined psychotherapy as augmentation to antidepressant treatment[37, 40-42] and two studies examined psychotherapy as substitution treatment.[37, 49] The STAR*D trial reflects the greatest ecological validity of the studies reviewed, because it accounted for patient preference in randomization and is most reflective of treatment provided in primary care settings. One study suggested that psychotherapy used as augmentation had better impact on clinical symptoms of MDD than medication alone[41] whereas Kennedy et al. found the opposite effect.[42] The remaining studies did not detect any difference between psychotherapy augmentation and continuation on antidepressant treatment.[37, 40] Substitution of antidepressant therapy with psychotherapy appeared to have the same benefit as substituting another antidepressant[37] or continuing previous medication.[49] While each of the studies included in this review addressed at least a portion of the initial key research question, none of the studies provides a complete answer to the initial question nor does an amalgamated consideration of the studies provide an entirely sufficient answer to the initial question. Most studies appeared to be underpowered to detect moderately large treatment effects, and conclusions are tempered by the heterogeneity in study designs and patient populations and limited number of good quality trials. We conclude that although current trials do not support favoring psychotherapy over antidepressant medication for mid-life adults with treatment resistant MDD, psychotherapy appears to be an equally effective treatment compared to antidepressant medication and is therefore a reasonable treatment option for this demographic. Whether these results are directly applicable to Veterans is uncertain. Veterans are on average older and have high rates of psychiatric and medical co-morbidity, clinical characteristics that were not well described in the studies reviewed.

Treatment via psychotherapy continues to face numerous barriers both in primary care and specialty mental health settings. The first consideration is access to psychotherapy. Many Veterans live in underserved areas and may have to travel farther to access facilities that would offer psychotherapeutic interventions. This issue is exacerbated by the greater time commitment required to receive traditional psychotherapy, which often requires weekly or biweekly face-to-face contact for an hour each. A second consideration is the relative cost of delivering psychotherapy versus providing antidepressant medications. The baseline costs of psychotherapy are typically higher, especially when delivered by a mental health professional such as a psychologist.[50, 51] However, there appears to be dispute when mid to long-term outcomes are measured. Some studies have demonstrated that antidepressant medications are more cost-effective within 1 year of follow-up for both direct and indirect costs.[52, 53], whereas other studies have not found differences in direct, aggregate or societal costs.[51, 54, 55] Studies have found psychotherapy to be superior in reducing costs related to missed work [56], treatment of medical comorbidities[57], and relapse.[45] Therefore, the cost-benefit ratio of antidepressant treatment versus psychotherapy remains disputed. A further limitation is that no current study has examined the cost-effectiveness of the two treatments in patients who do not respond to initial antidepressant treatment. Because TRD is both common and costly[58], large, high quality, long-term randomized trials are needed to evaluate the effectiveness and cost-effectiveness of different treatment strategies for patients with TRD.

One strategy to increase access and cost-effectiveness of psychotherapy involves collaborative care. Recent research has shown that training non-mental health professionals (e.g., nurses) to provide brief psychotherapeutic interventions are effective in reducing depressive symptoms.[59-61] Collaborative care models involving depression care managers has been shown to improve the quality of depression care, symptom severity, patient satisfaction, and functional impairment.[50, 62] Some of these trials[59, 63] utilized empirically based psychotherapy as a step-2 treatment option for treatment resistant patients. These studies were conducted in older adults with MDD or dysthymia who are more similar to the Veteran population than most of the studies we reviewed in the current evidence synthesis. Unfortunately, the psychotherapy was delivered as part of a package of collaborative care and its unique contribution to improved outcomes cannot be assessed. Nevertheless, evidence suggests that training non-mental health professionals to deliver brief psychotherapy may improve outcomes in primary care patients without burdening resources within the VA system.

Prior systematic reviews [19-23] have shown that psychotherapy and antidepressant medications have similar benefit in acute phase treatment for MDD. For patients with chronic MDD or dysthymia, current evidence supports the combination of psychotherapy and antidepressant medication for initial treatment. Treatment resistant depression is common and a greater number of effective treatment options are needed. Our evidence synthesis found only limited studies that do not support psychotherapy as a step-2 strategy, either for augmentation or as a substitute for antidepressant medication.

LIMITATIONS

Several limitations of the current literature emerged upon review. First, few RCTs exist that adequately address the question of resistant depression. In the future, this may be addressed in two ways: 1) re-analysis of existing data from trials in which patients with TRD are recruited, or 2) conducting studies designed to examine this question. Second, there was significant heterogeneity in how resistant depression was defined in the different studies. Measures included interviewer rated depression scales (e.g., HAM-D), self-report depression scales (e.g., BDI), DSM diagnostic criteria (DSM-III-R or DSM-IV), and clinical judgment. Future studies should consider a standardized operational definition of TRD to facilitate comparisons across studies. Third, all of the studies involved comparators that received active treatment. True placebo controlled trials may be necessary to compare the relative effects of psychotherapy and antidepressants as second step treatments. Fourth, none of the six studies reviewed involved patients from within the VA. Compared to the general population, Veterans have higher incidences of depression with psychiatric and medical comorbidities.[4] Therefore, results of the current review may have limited generalizability to the VA population. Fifth, only two psychotherapeutic strategies have been considered in the limited literature, with the majority using CT. Traditionally, CT requires a minimum of 12-16 sessions and is often delivered by trained experts. As a result, none of the psychotherapies reviewed were likely to be administered within the primary care setting. This is in contrast with the larger literature, where brief therapies such as problem-solving therapy and interpersonal therapy have been adapted by non-mental health professionals with demonstrated improvements as first step treatments in primary care settings.[50] Studies to compare the effectiveness of differing psychotherapies could inform policy.

FUTURE RESEARCH

There is a pressing need to conduct RCTs examining psychotherapy as a second step treatment in patients who have not responded to initial antidepressant medication treatment. Studies conducted within the VA would provide the best evidence on how to treat veterans. As more OEF/OIF veterans return with significant medical and psychiatric comorbidities, this question will become critical in the management of MDD.

Future investigations should also address cost-effectiveness of the different treatment options. To our knowledge, no current study has examined the cost-effectiveness of psychotherapy versus antidepressant treatment when used as second step treatment. As a first step, analyses using observational data from the VA depression registry may be informative. Ideally, however, studies designed for this purpose would involve longer follow-up, as well as measures of direct costs, indirect costs, and costs associated with comorbid non-psychiatric conditions. Finally, innovative interventions are needed that adapt validated psychotherapeutic techniques to primary care settings. The VA has already initiated primary care mental health integration techniques; however, there remains a need for trials of depression treatments to inform the specific treatments offered in these integrated models. This will be crucial in improving access for underserved veterans while simultaneously reducing the strain on the VA resources.

APPENDIX A: SEARCH STRATEGY

**Question: In primary care patients with major depressive disorder who do not achieve
remission with acute phase antidepressant treatment, is empirically based psychotherapy
used as an augmentation or substitution treatment more effective than control for achieving
remission? Empirically based psychotherapies to be considered are: cognitive behavioral
therapy, interpersonal therapy, problem-solving therapy, dialectical behavior therapy, and
acceptance and commitment therapy.**

Inclusion Criteria- Systematic Reviews

Systematic Review

Does psychotherapy benefit patients who have been previously not responded to adequate
pharmacotherapy?

Search Strategy for Systematic Review: Database: **PubMed Medline** – 1950 to February 26, 2009

1	"Depressive Disorder"[Mesh] OR (major AND depression)	71993
2	((problem-solving OR interpersonal OR dialectical behav* OR acceptance OR commitment OR mindfulness) AND (therapy OR psychotherapy)) OR "Psychotherapy"[Mesh] OR "Behavior Therapy"[Mesh]	229473
3	("Combined Modality Therapy"[Mesh] OR Drug resistant[Mesh] OR additive OR augmentation OR augment* OR relaps* OR recurrent OR refractory OR resistant OR persisten* OR treatment failure[Mesh])	1147546
4	#1 AND #2 AND #3	1997
5	Limits: **Humans, English, All Adult: 19+ years**	1078
6	systematic[sb]	116759
7	#5 AND #6	34
8	Cochrane Database Syst Rev [TA] OR search[Title/Abstract] OR meta-analysis[Publication Type] OR MEDLINE[Title/abstract] OR (systematic[Title/Abstract] AND review[Title/Abstract])	140388
9	#5 AND #8	24
10	#7 OR #9	41

For Systematic Reviews, the Medline search yielded 41 articles. Title and abstracts were
reviewed by 2 independent persons who identified 12 articles for full text review. Of the 12
reviewed, 0 were identified as meeting the inclusion criteria previously established; therefore no
systematic reviews will be included for this question in the final report.

Inclusion Criteria- Randomized Controlled Trials

Randomized controlled trials

Outpatient setting

Patients from general population (not special populations)

Adults who have not remised or responded significantly to anti-depressant medication for > 6 wks and not in therapy (CBT, IPT, Sol. Focused, DBT, ACT, MBT)

If mixed sample, at least 80% must be partial or non-responders or outcomes reported separately

Exclude: patients with MDD where guidelines recommend mental health specialty care (eg. high suicidality, substance abuse, borderline personality d/o)

Relevant comparison

English language articles

Search Strategy for Randomized Controlled Trials: Database: **PubMed Medline** - 1950 to February 26, 2009

1	"Depressive Disorder"[Mesh] OR (major AND depression)	71993
2	((problem-solving OR interpersonal OR dialectical behav* OR acceptance OR commitment OR mindfulness) AND (therapy OR psychotherapy)) OR "Psychotherapy"[Mesh] OR "Behavior Therapy"[Mesh]	229441
3	"Combined Modality Therapy"[Mesh] OR Drug resistant[Mesh] OR additive OR augmentation OR augment* OR relaps* OR recurrent OR refractory OR resistant OR persisten* OR treatment failure[Mesh]	1147546
4	randomized controlled trial[Publication Type] OR (randomized[Title/Abstract] AND controlled[Title/Abstract] AND trial[Title/Abstract])	275228
5	#1 AND #2 AND #3 AND #4	422
6	Limits: Humans, English, All Adult: 19+ years	333

For Randomized Control Trials, the Medline search yielded 333 articles. Title and abstracts were reviewed by 2 independent persons who identified 43 articles for full text review. Of the 43 articles reviewed, 12 were identified as meeting the inclusion criteria previously established.

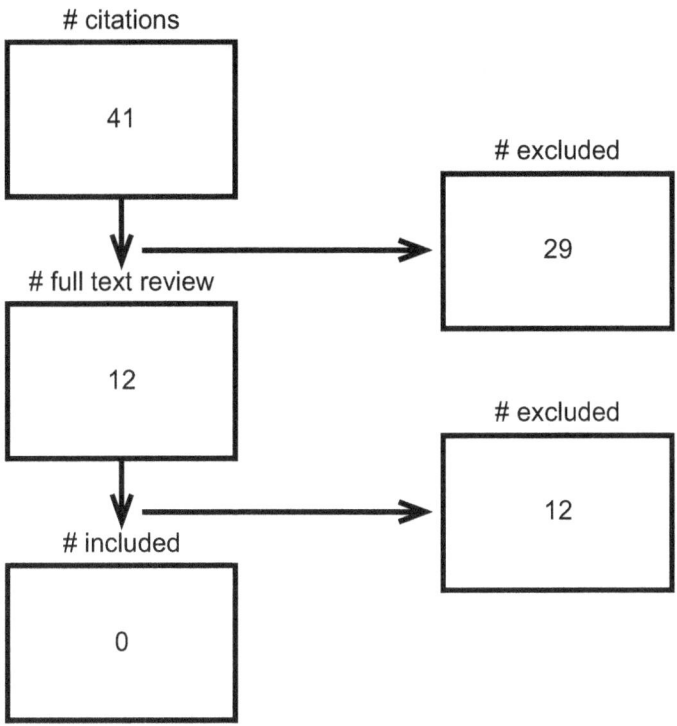

Figure 1. Systematic Reviews Literature Flow

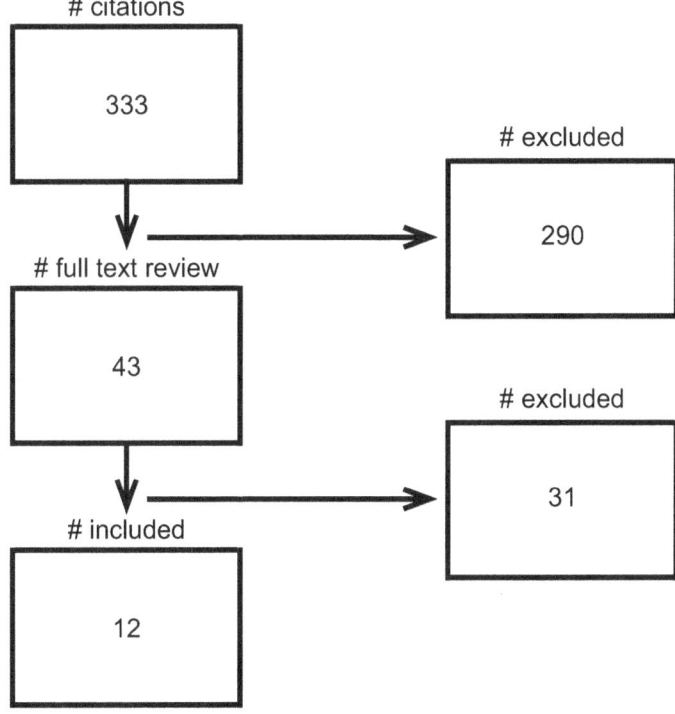

Figure 2. Randomized Controlled Trials Literature Flow

APPENDIX B: PEER REVIEW

Question 1: Are the objectives, scope, and methods for this review clearly described?

Reviewer	Comment	Reply
1	Excellent description of objectives, scope, and methods. This review exposes the scarcity of good studies to answer this question. The conclusions fit the data.	Acknowledged
2	Clearly described, concisely written, comprehensive, well thought out review.	Acknowledged
3	The authors have been particularly thorough in describing clearly the objectives, scope, and methods for this review. I don't believe any reader would be left with any question about these. (As a small matter, on page 15, "solution-focused therapy" was listed as one of the empirically-based psychotherapies that were considered for purposes of the study. However, in Appendix A, this was not listed as one of the search terms; "problem-solving" was listed. I think these are both terms of art, and are different. Do you want to conform the terms? I think the authors likely considered problem solving therapy, but not solution-focused therapy.)	Acknowledged Thank you for pointing out this discrepancy. We have now changed the term "solution-focused therapy" to "problem-solving therapy" to reflect terms included in the literature search (pg 15, 16).

Question 2: Is there any indication of bias in our synthesis of the evidence?

Reviewer	Comment	Reply
1	No indication of bias. This review follows rigorous methods for systematic selection and analysis	Acknowledged
2	No	Acknowledged
3	I see no indication of bias in the synthesis of the evidence. Indeed, it appears that the authors have gone out of their way to eliminate any opportunity for bias.	Acknowledged

Question 3 Are there any studies on responsiveness of depression questionnaires or relapse prevention trials related to this report that we have overlooked?

Reviewer	Comment	Reply
1	I don't know of any others	Acknowledged
2	None	Acknowledged
3	I don't know of any studies on the effectiveness of psychotherapy as a second step treatment for MDD in patients who do not achieve remission after initial treatment with antidepressants, per se, that have been overlooked.	Acknowledged

Question 4: Please write additional suggestions or additional comments below for this report. If applicable, please indicate the page and line numbers from the draft report.

Reviewer	Comment	Reply
1	P 6, last line: suggest changing "control" to "comparison group," a term that is more consistent with most patients in this group being on some form of treatment. This review achieves impressive rigor and thoroughness for such a limited number of studies.	We agree with this assertion and have attempted to make this point throughout the review. However, in that specific place, we have opted to retain the wording as initially developed by VA Central Office to avoid confusion regarding the question we were originally attempting to answer with this review.

2	**4.**	
	a. p. 9 typo, 2nd line from bottom: should be "antidepressant medication *with* CT.	a. Thank you for finding this error. The typo has been corrected.
	b. p.10 I think the summary and conclusions understate the equivalence of CT vs medication as a switch choice. The STAR*D data suggested little difference for the between CT and meds for the switch arms, and hence for patients who would prefer CT it may be a reasonable option. c. I'm concerned with the statement: "Based on this sparse evidence, we conclude that current trials do not support a benefit from adding psychotherapy to antidepressant medication for mid-life adults with treatment resistant MDD". While it is technically correct, I think it is at risk of being mis-interpreted too strongly as an indication that there is no role for CT as an adjunct in TRD. It seems the evidence is insufficient to conclude one way or the other, and I think the wording should reflect that the current data do not support a benefit, but that the data is insufficient to make a conclusion and that future studies may likely change this result.	b.& c. We agree with the reviewer that our summary and conclusions did not emphasize the equivalence of the two treatment modalities. We have modified the summary statements on pages 9, 10, and 30 to reflect the equivalence that we generally observed in studies comparing CT and meds, and to reflect our belief that CT remains a reasonable treatment option in patients with TRD. As we state repeatedly in the review, the current evidence is not sufficient to determine the superiority of one treatment modality over the other. Future research with rigorous study designs is necessary to definitively answer this question.
	d. p.20. Table 1 might benefit from a row that allows a better comparison of the level of depressive severity when beginning psychotherapy treatment, for e.g., clarifying the BDI or QIDS scores as "mild", "moderate" or "severe", and a row that allows comparison of the prior antidepressant treatment (e.g., antidepressant type, dose, duration). Also, can one report the number of prior treatment failures for the current episode? Finally, the definition of persistent depression (listed in the evidence tables in the appendices) is quite information and would be a useful row in Table 1. I realize, however, that some of this information may not be available for many studies.	d. Per the reviewer's suggestion, we report that that depression severity in each study was "moderate." We agree with the reviewer that the number of failures of treatment may be important information in evaluating the extent of TRD; however, this information was not reported in the reviewed studies and hence cannot be included. We agree that describing persistent depression within the text would be helpful. We have incorporated this suggestion by creating a new table (Table 2) that describes the various definitions of persistent depression, and summarizes antidepressant type, dosage, and duration. The Additional information about prior antidepressant treatment was also added to the definitions of persistent depression in the evidence tables in the appendices.
	e. Can the authors clarify whether any of the studies directly addressed the research question they pose? If not, how might they suggest designing a future research project to address this question directly? Also, might they suggest a study to address the long term risk benefits of a switch to CT (or an empirically based psychotherapy) vs medications?	e. A sentence was added to the discussion on page 30 clarifying our position that we do not consider the initial key research question adequately answered by our review. Regarding the reviewer's suggestion of designing a study, our current (cont'd.)

2 (cont'd)		version outlines important components of such a study in the Future Research section (pg 35) as well as highlights these in the Summary and Discussion section. Specifically, we highlight the need to study TRD in the context of impact on work, medical comorbidities, relapse, and the need for cost-effectiveness analysis of the different treatments available.
3	This report looked at the *condition* of treatment resistant major depression that failed to respond to an adequate dose of antidepressant treatment. I wonder if it would be worth looking at *individuals* who have treatment resistant major depression that failed to respond to an adequate dose of antidepressant treatment? I know of two recent studies that may be worth reviewing: Watchful waiting for minor depression in primary care: remission rates and predictors of improvement. M.T. Hegel et al. General Hospital Psychiatry 28 (2006) 205–212. This study suggests that for treatment-seeking samples with minor depression in primary care an avoidant coping style seriously interferes with remission, and engaging in regular active pleasant events confers an advantage. It further suggests that feasible interventions for primary care that promote activity and decrease avoidant coping styles may improve outcomes. Cortico-limbic response to personally challenging emotional stimuli after complete recovery from depression. J.M. Hooley et al. Psychiatry Research: Neuroimaging 171 (2009) 106–119. This study suggests that vulnerability to depression may be associated with abnormalities in cortico-limbic activation that are independent of mood state and that remain even after full recovery. Perhaps there are similar processes at work in those with treatment resistant major depression that failed to respond to an adequate dose of antidepressant treatment that would not respond to traditional psychotherapeutic approaches.	The reviewer makes an interesting point. The Hegel study suggests that patients with minor depression may be successfully treated in primary care through pleasant activities and by reducing avoidant coping. The extensive literature on coping and depression supports this conclusion. It is likely that patients with minor depression may be patients who have residual symptoms after an MDD episode, in other words, TRD. However, it seems that a discussion of such interventions is beyond the scope of this review because of our original goal of comparing CT with medications in a treatment resistant population. Future reviews may address this issue by incorporating all treatments provided in primary care settings, and treatments provided to patients who may or may not have TRD. Regarding the Hooley study, it would be certainly worthwhile to determine the neurological mechanisms that may contribute to TRD and/or relapse. Unfortunately, a discussion of such mechanisms is beyond the scope of this review as defined by the VA Central office.

Question 5: Recommendations for future ESP topical areas of interest or programmatic comments may also be included at the end of this section.

Reviewer	Comment	Reply
1	No comment	Acknowledged
2	None	
3	I agree wholeheartedly with the statement on page 34 that there remains a need for trials of depression treatments to inform the specific treatments offered (and to be offered) in primary care mental health integration models. This is a pressing need. I would argue that the population of patients that could benefit from efficacious and effective treatments in such models is far larger than the population of patients who suffer from treatment resistant depression.	Acknowledged

APPENDIX C: EVIDENCE TABLES OF RCTS

Evidence Synthesis for Determining the Efficacy of Psychotherapy for Treatment Resistant Depression

Study ID	Persistence Definition & Treatments	Study Information	Participants	Results	Comments/Quality Scoring
Harley et al., 2008	**Persistent Depression:** Despite stable, adequate medication treatment for MDD (as determined by consensus of 2 senior psychiatrists with expertise in MDD), patients still met criteria for MDD on the SCID-I.	**Geographical location:** Boston, MA	**Age:** [mean] Total: 41.8	**1) Interviewer rated depression severity:**	**Comments:** Small sample sizes, limited information provided on samples' baseline characteristics, and confound of individual therapy.
		Setting: MHC; participants were referred by outpatient providers.	**Sex:** [female %] Total: 75%	**HAM-D at baseline:** [mean (SD)] DBT: 16.15 (4.47) WL: 18.64 (4.72)	**Quality assessment:**
		VA sites: No	**Race/ethnicity:** [white (%)] Total: 83%	**HAM-D at follow-up:** [mean (SD)] DBT: 11.30 (5.31) WL: 17.11 (6.23)	Randomization adequate?: Y Allocation concealment adequate?: Y Baseline comparability?: Y
	Psychotherapy: Dialectical Behavior Therapy (DBT) Group DBT based depression skills group; 16 weekly sessions lasting 90 minutes each.	**Study design:** RCT	**Duration of current episode in days:** [mean (SD)] DBT: 201.00 (131.59) WL: 292.40 (374.94)	*DBT group had significantly lower HAM-D scores than WL (F=4.63; p<.05; D=1.45).*	Valid outcome assessment?: Y Subject/providers blind?: N Outcomes assessed blind?: Y Dropout rate < 30%?: Y Differential dropout rate < 10%?: Y
		Number of participants enrolled: Total: 24 DBT: 13 WL: 11	**Number of lifetime antidepressant trials:** [mean (SD)] DBT: 3.31 (1.70) WL: 4.27 (2.45)	**2) Self-reported depression severity:**	Incomplete data addressed adequately?: Unknown Conflict of interest?: N
		Duration of follow up: 16 weeks	**Number of hospitalizations:** [mean (SD)] DBT: 0.85 (0.99) WL: 0.27 (0.65)	**BDI at baseline:** [mean (SD)] DBT: 27.31 (8.83) WL: 27.44 (11.66)	Overall quality rating: Fair
	Comparator: Wait List (WL) Pts in this group continued treatment as usual, which included taking prescribed medications and meeting with psychiatrists and other providers as usual.	**Inclusion criteria:** - Age 18-65 - Principal diagnosis of MDD on SCID - Have an established treatment relationship with a psychiatrist - Stabilized on adequate dose of antidepressant medication before entering study (no dosage change for at least 6 weeks before study entry)	**Age at first MDE:** [mean (SD)] DBT: 27.08 (14.23) WL: 25.18 (15.20)	**BDI at follow-up:** [mean (SD)] DBT: 15.10 (12.13) WL: 25.89 (16.30)	
		Exclusion criteria: - Bipolar disorder - Psychotic spectrum disorders - Active substance abuse or dependence - Mental retardation - Pervasive developmental disorder - Active suicidality - Severe or unstable medical conditions - Patients with previous or current CBT experience - Borderline Personality Disorder	**Engaged in concurrent non-CBT individual therapy:** Total: 83%	*DBT group had significantly lower BDI scores than WL (F=9.50; p<.01; D=1.31).*	

Study ID	Persistence Definition & Treatments	Study Information	Participants	Results	Comments/Quality Scoring
Kennedy et al., 2003	**Persistent depression:** Having initially met criteria for MDE with HAM-D-17≥16 and after 8-14 weeks of antidepressant treatment with moclobemide (300-600 mg/day), paroxetine (20-40 mg/day), sertraline (50-200 mg/day), or venlafaxine (75-225 mg/day), patients still had HAM-D=8-15. **Psychotherapy:** <u>Cognitive Therapy (CT)</u> 12 sessions over 8 weeks in combination with AD therapy; pts were also seen every 4 weeks for a medication check up. **Comparator:** <u>Lithium Augmentation (LA)</u> Pts who were considered "partial responders" had their AD therapy augmented with 600 mg/day of lithium carbonate, which clinicians could increase by 300 mg/ day after 2-4 weeks. Pts were seen every 2 weeks for routine clinical management.	**Geographical location:** Toronto, Canada **Setting:** MHC **VA sites:** No **Study design:** RCT **Number of participants enrolled:** Total: 44 CT: 23 LA: 21 **Duration of follow up:** 8 weeks **Inclusion criteria:** - Age 18-65 - Partial response after receiving maximum tolerated doses of moclobemide, paroxetine, sertraline, or venlafaxine (choice of antidepressant was at the discretion of the treating psychiatrist) for 8-14 weeks - Initially met criteria for MDE - HAM-D-17≥16 - At least one prior MDE **Exclusion criteria:** - Major medical disorder - Organic brain syndrome - Schizophrenia or schizoaffective disorder - Bipolar disorder - MDD with psychotic features - Substance or alcohol use or dependence within past 6 months	**Age:** [mean (SD)] CT: 40.7 (12.5) LA: 37.7 (11.3) **Sex:** [female, n (%)] CT: 12 (52.2%) LA: 12 (57%) **Race/ethnicity:** Not reported **Duration of current episode in weeks:** [mean (SD)] CT: 126.4 (170.4) LA: 119.8 (160.8) **Number of prior episodes:** [mean (SD)] CT: 2.1 (1.5) LA: 2.3 (1.4) **Age at first MDE:** [mean (SD)] CT: 26.3 (13.5) LA: 24.4 (13.6) **Comorbid psychiatric diagnoses:** [n (%)] CT: 8 (35%) LA: 4 (19%)	**1) Interviewer rated depression severity:** **HAM-D-17 after 8-14 weeks med treatment:** [mean (SD)] CT: 12.1 (2.2) LA: 11.6 (1.9) **HAM-D-17 at follow-up:** [mean (SD)] CT: 14.8 (9.9) LA: 9.2 (6.7) *LA group had significantly lower HAM-D-17 scores than CT group in intent-to-treat analysis (t=2.02; df=42; p=.04; d=.32).* **2) Self-reported depression severity:** **BDI after 8-14 weeks med treatment:** [mean (SD)] CT: 22.7 (8.6) LA: 22.4 (10.3) **BDI at follow-up:** [mean (SD)] CT: 19.9 (10.3) LA: 15.1 (11.4) *No significant differences between groups.*	**Comments:** Only included partial responders; excluded non-responders. **Quality assessment:** Randomization adequate?: Y Allocation concealment adequate?: Y Baseline comparability?: Y Valid outcome assessment?: Y Subject/providers blind?: N Outcomes assessed blind?: Y Dropout rate < 30%?: Y Differential dropout rate < 10%?: Y Incomplete data addressed adequately?: Y Conflict of interest?: N Overall quality rating: Good

Evidence Synthesis for Determining the Efficacy of Psychotherapy for Treatment Resistant Depression

Study ID	Persistence Definition & Treatments	Study Information	Participants	Results	Comments/Quality Scoring
Paykel et al., 1999 Paykel et al., 2005 Scott et al., 2003 Scott et al., 2000* Teasdale et al., 2001 *Data were primarily extracted from this reference.	**Persistent depression:** Despite treatment with tricyclic antidepressant, SSRI, atypical AD, or MAOI for at least 8 weeks (with 4 or more weeks of minimum dosage equivalent to at least 125 mg of amitriptyline), patients still had HAM-D≥8 & BDI≥9. **Psychotherapy:** <u>Cognitive Therapy (CT)</u> 16 sessions over 20 weeks. Pts also received CM. **Comparator:** <u>Clinical Management (CM)</u> Antidepressant continuation; pts seen every 4 weeks during tx and every 8 weeks during follow-up for 30 minutes each.	**Geographical location:** Cambridge & Newcastle, England **Setting:** MHC; Psychiatric Outpatient Clinics **VA sites:** No **Study design:** RCT **Number of participants enrolled:** Total: 158 CT: 80 CMT: 78 **Duration of follow up:** 20 weeks **Inclusion criteria:** - Age 21-65 - DSM-III-R MDD within past 18 months but not MDD criteria in past 2 months & HRSD ≥ 8 & BDI ≥ 9. **Exclusion criteria:** - Bipolar disorder - Cyclothymia - Schizoaffective disorder - Drug or alcohol dependence - Antisocial behavior or self-harm - Dysthymia before age 20 - Borderline personality - Learning disability - Organic brain damage - Other primary Axis I disorder - Currently receiving psychotherapy or previously received CT for more than 5 sessions	**Age:** [mean (SD)] CT: 43.5 (9.8) CM: 43.2 (11.2) **Sex:** [female, n (%)] CT: 37 (46%) CM: 41 (53%) **Race/ethnicity:** Not reported **Duration of depressive episode in months:** [median (1st & 3rd quartiles)] CT: 14.5 (9, 18) CTM: 13 (9, 21) **Prior episodes of MDD:** [median (1st & 3rd quartiles)] CT: 2 (1, ≥3) CM: 2 (1, ≥3)	1) **Interviewer rated depression severity:** **HDRS baseline after 8 week drug trial:** [mean (SD)] CT=12.1 (2.7) CM=12.2 (2.9) **HDRS at follow-up:** [mean (SD)] CT=8.7 (5.3) CM=9.4 (5.3) *No significant between group differences or group x time interactions over 20 week treatment phase or 68 week follow-up (F=2.2; df=1324; p=.14)* 2) **Self-reported depression severity:** **BDI baseline after 8 week drug trial:** [mean (SD)] CT=21.7 (7.7) CM= 22.3 (8.0) **BDI at follow-up:** [mean (SD)] CT=13.8 (9.6) CM= 16.1 (10.0) *No significant between group differences or group x time interactions over 20 week treatment phase or 68 week follow-up (F=2.3; df=1293; p=.13)*	**Comments:** Not currently depressed; partially remitted but with residual symptoms - because not MDD but still some depressive symptoms on HDRS and BDI In Scott et al. 2000, found that some dep sx showed sig effects on drug refractory residual symptoms Both CT and CM led to improvement in dep sx **Quality assessment:** Randomization adequate?: Y Allocation concealment adequate?: Y Baseline comparability?: Y Valid outcome assessment?: Y Subject/providers blind?: N/Y Outcomes assessed blind?: Y Dropout rate < 30%?: Y Differential dropout rate < 10%?: Y Incomplete data addressed adequately?: Y Conflict of interest?: N Overall quality rating: Good

28

Evidence Synthesis for Determining the Efficacy of Psychotherapy for Treatment Resistant Depression

Study ID	Persistence Definition & Treatments	Study Information	Participants	Results	Comments/Quality Scoring
Rush et al., 2004 Rush et al., 2006 Thase et al., 2007* Wisniewski et al., 2007 STAR*D *Data were primarily extracted from this reference.	**Persistent depression:** Following treatment with citalopram (20 mg/day to start, 40 mg/day by week 4, and maximum potential dosage of 60 mg/day by week 6) for 14 weeks, patients still had HAM-D≥14. **Psychotherapy:** Cognitive Therapy (CT) 16 sessions delivered twice weekly for weeks 1-4, then once weekly for 8 remaining weeks. *Switch to CT:* Pts discontinued citalopram and began CT. *Augment CT:* Pts continued on citalopram and added CT. **Comparator:** Antidepressant Medication (ADM) *Switch ADM:* Pts discontinued citalopram and began bupropion, sertraline, or venlafaxine. *Augment ADM:* Pts continued on citalopram and added bupropion or buspirone.	**Geographical location:** 14 Regional centers across TX, MA, NY, PA, OK, KS, CA: LA and San Diego, NC, IL, MI, VA, TN, AL **Setting:** 18-Primary Care, 23 MHC **VA sites:** No **Study design:** randomized multi-step clinical trial **Number of participants enrolled:** Total: 304 Switch to CT=36 Augment CT=65 Switch ADM=86 Augment ADM=117 **Duration of follow up:** 14 weeks **Inclusion criteria:** - Age 18-75 - Non psychotic MDD - HRSD17≥14 **Exclusion criteria:** - Bipolar, schizophrenia, eating d/o, OCD - Hx of intolerability or resistance to ≥1 Anti-dep with adequate dosage - ≥7 days Citalopram use prior to study enrollment - non-responsive ≥16 session of CT in current MDD episode - Medical contraindication - Pregnant females - Requires psychiatric hospitalization, antipsychotics, or mood stabilizers	**Age:** [mean (SD)] Switch to CT: 43.4 (14.7) Augment CT: 40.6 (11.5) Switch ADM=41.5 (13.3) Augment ADM=39.7 (13.5) **Sex:** [female, n (%)] Switch to CT: 22 (61.1%) Augment CT: 41 (63.1%) Switch ADM: 53 (61.6%) Augment ADM: 78 (66.7%) **Race/ethnicity:** [white, n (%)] Switch to CT: 28 (77.8%) Augment CT: 52 (80.0%) Switch ADM: 63 (73.3%) Augment ADM: 99 (84.6%) **Duration of depressive episode in months:** [mean (SD)] Switch to CT: 17.4 (31.2) Augment CT: 29.6 (49.4) Switch ADM: 26.5 (54.0) Augment ADM: 20.0 (47.5) **Number of prior episodes of MDD:** [mean (SD)] Switch to CT: 8.7 (18.8) Augment CT: 7.3 (14.1) Switch ADM: 8.4 (16.0) Augment ADM: 4.6 (5.4)	**1) Interviewer rated depression severity:** **HRSD at start of Level 2:** [mean (SD)] Switch to CT: 16.4 (6.2) Augment CT: 17.8 (5.7) Switch ADM: 17.7 (6.6) Augment ADM: 16.0 (6.7) **Met remission criteria on (HRSD≤7) at end of Level 2:** Switch to CT: 25.0% Augment CT: 23.1% Switch ADM: 27.9% Augment ADM: 33.3% *No significant differences between groups.* **2) Self-reported depression severity:** **QIDS-C at start of Level 2:** [mean (SD)] Switch to CT: 11.2 (4.3) Augment CT: 11.9 (4.3) Switch ADM: 12.1 (4.6) Augment ADM: 12.0 (4.6) **QIDS-C at end of Level 2:** [mean (SD)] Switch to CT: 9.1 (5.4) Augment CT: 8.2 (5.1) Switch ADM: 9.1 (5.0) Augment ADM: 8.2 (4.8) *No significant differences between groups.*	**Comments:** Due to equipoise-stratified randomization, <1/3 agreed to randomization. Low rates of psychotherapy acceptability are at odds with real world experience of the STAR*D authors. Baseline differences in Augment CT more impaired & lower QOL than Augment ADM and Switch to CT lower income than Switch ADM. Numerous pharmaceutical companies supported the project. **Quality assessment:** Randomization adequate?: Y/N Allocation concealment adequate?: Y Baseline comparability?: Y/N Valid outcome assessment?: Y Subject/providers blind?: N Outcomes assessed blind?: Y Dropout rate < 30%?: Y Differential dropout rate < 10%?: Y Incomplete data addressed adequately?: Y Conflict of interest?: Y Overall quality rating: Good

Evidence Synthesis for Determining the Efficacy of Psychotherapy for Treatment Resistant Depression

Study ID	Persistence Definition & Treatments	Study Information	Participants*	Results	Comments/Quality Scoring
Blackburn & Moore, 1997	**Persistent depression:** Despite showing significant reduction in depressive symptoms over 16 weeks of treatment with antidepressant medication of the general practitioner's choice (prescribed at or above therapeutic doses), patients on average continued to have depressive symptoms in the moderate range on the BDI and above the traditional cut point of 11 on the HAM-D. **Psychotherapy:** Cognitive Therapy (CT) 27 sessions delivered over 2 years, with pts being seen 3 times in 1st month, twice in 2nd month, and monthly thereafter. **Comparator:** Antidepressant Medication (ADM) Maintenance ADM was of general practitioner's choice (tricyclics, MAOIs, SSRIs), as long as prescribed at or above recognized maintenance dose.	**Geographical location:** Scotland **Setting:** MHC; participants were recruited from outpatient referrals to consultants in a large teaching psychiatric hospital and from 2 general practices. **VA sites:** No **Study design:** RCT **Number of participants enrolled:** Total: 37 (48 initially) CT: 17 (22 initially) ADM: 20 (26 initially) **Duration of follow up:** 24 months **Inclusion criteria:** - Age 18-65 - Diagnosis of primary major unipolar depression, non-psychotic - Score of at least 16 on HRSD - Current episode had to be at least second MDE **Exclusion criteria:** - Having another primary Axis I disorder - Organic brain damage - History of bipolar illness - Alcohol or drug misuse - Could not be prescribed antidepressant medication for medical reasons - Unwilling to be randomly allocated to treatment	**Age:** [mean (SD)] CT: 37.8 (13.1) ADM: 40.1 (12.7) **Sex:** [female, n (%)] CT: 17/22 (77%) ADM: 17/26 (65%) **Race/ethnicity:** Not given **Duration of current episode in months:** [mean (SD)] CT: 7.0 (1.4) ADM: 6.9 (1.3) **Number of prior episodes:** [mean (SD)] CT: 4.1 (3.4) ADM: 3.2 (2.2) **Number of hospitalizations:** [mean (SD)] CT: 0.7 (0.9) ADM: 0.8 (2.3) **Number of suicide attempts:** [mean (SD)] CT: 0.4 (0.7) ADM: 0.9 (1.9) *Data based on initially enrolled participants.	**1) Interviewer rated depression severity:** **HRSD baseline after 16 weeks acute med treatment:** [mean (SD)] CT: 11.8 (6.3) ADM: 10.6 (6.8) **HRSD interpolated over 24 months follow-up:** [mean (SD)] CT: 8.6 (5.6) ADM: 9.3 (7.2) *ANCOVA showed no significant difference between treatments (F=0.31; d.f.=2, 55; NS).* **2) Self-reported depression severity:** **BDI baseline after 16 weeks acute med treatment:** [mean (SD)] CT: 20.4 (11.1) ADM: 19.7 (14.2) **BDI interpolated over 24 months follow-up:** [mean (SD)] CT: 14.2 (9.9) ADM: 18.1 (13.1) *ANCOVA showed no significant difference between treatments (F=0.72; d.f.=2, 53; NS).*	**Comments:** Reviewers decided based on data after 16 weeks of treatment that samples met criteria for persistent depression. ANCOVAs compared 3 groups, not just the 2 groups of interest. 35% retention for CT and 25% retention for ADM. **Quality assessment:** Randomization adequate?: Y Allocation concealment adequate?: Y Baseline comparability?: Y Valid outcome assessment?: Y Subject/providers blind?: N Outcomes assessed blind?: Y Dropout rate < 30%?: N Differential dropout rate < 10%?: N Incomplete data addressed adequately?: Y Conflict of interest?: N Overall quality rating: Poor

REFERENCES

1.   Papakostas G, Fava M. Predictors, moderators, and mediators (correlates) of treatment outcome in major depressive disorder. Dialogues in Clinical Neuroscience. 2008;10(4):439-451.

2.   Hasin DS, Goodwin RD, Stinson FS, Grant BF. Epidemiology of major depressive disorder: results from the National Epidemiologic Survey on Alcoholism and Related Conditions. Arch Gen Psychiatry. 2005;62(10):1097-106.

3.   Kessler RC, Berglund P, Demler O, Jin R, Merikangas KR, Walters EE. Lifetime prevalence and age-of-onset distributions of DSM-IV disorders in the National Comorbidity Survey Replication. Arch Gen Psychiatry. 2005;62(6):593-602.

4.   Hankin CS, Spiro A, 3rd, Miller DR, Kazis L. Mental disorders and mental health treatment among U.S. Department of Veterans Affairs outpatients: the Veterans Health Study. Am J Psychiatry. 1999;156(12):1924-30.

5.   Katon WJ. Clinical and health services relationships between major depression, depressive symptoms, and general medical illness. Biol Psychiatry. 2003;54(3):216-26.

6.   Kessler RC, Berglund P, Demler O, et al. The epidemiology of major depressive disorder: results from the National Comorbidity Survey Replication (NCS-R). Jama. 2003;289(23):3095-105.

7.   Kronish IM, Rieckmann N, Halm EA, et al. Persistent depression affects adherence to secondary prevention behaviors after acute coronary syndromes. J Gen Intern Med. 2006;21(11):1178-83.

8.   Seelig MD, Katon W. Gaps in depression care: why primary care physicians should hone their depression screening, diagnosis, and management skills. J Occup Environ Med. 2008;50(4):451-8.

9.   Olfson M, Marcus SC, Druss B, Elinson L, Tanielian T, Pincus HA. National trends in the outpatient treatment of depression. JAMA. 2002;287(2):203-9.

10.   Karasu TB, Gelenberg A, Merriam A, Wang P. *Practice guideline for the treatment of patients with major depressive disorder.* 2nd ed Arlington, VA: American Psychiatric Association; 2000 APA Practice Guidelines).

11.   Fochtmann LJ, Gelenberg AJ. *Guideline watch: Practice guideline for the treatment of patients with depressive disorder.* 2nd ed Arlington, VA: American Psychiatric Association; 2005 APA Practice Guidelines).

12.   Barbui C, Furukawa TA, Cipriani A. Effectiveness of paroxetine in the treatment of acute major depression in adults: a systematic re-examination of published and unpublished data from randomized trials. Cmaj. 2008;178(3):296-305.

13. Cipriani A, Furukawa TA, Geddes JR, et al. Does randomized evidence support sertraline as first-line antidepressant for adults with acute major depression? A systematic review and meta-analysis. J Clin Psychiatry. 2008;69(11):1732-42.

14. Kennedy SH, Andersen HF, Thase ME. Escitalopram in the treatment of major depressive disorder: a meta-analysis. Curr Med Res Opin. 2009;25(1):161-75.

15. Mulrow CD, Williams JW, Jr., Chiquette E, et al. Efficacy of newer medications for treating depression in primary care patients. Am J Med. 2000;108(1):54-64.

16. Watanabe N, Omori IM, Nakagawa A, et al. Mirtazapine versus other antidepressants in the acute-phase treatment of adults with major depression: systematic review and meta-analysis. J Clin Psychiatry. 2008;69(9):1404-15.

17. Simon GE, Ludman E, Unutzer J, Bauer MS. Design and implementation of a randomized trial evaluating systematic care for bipolar disorder. Bipolar Disord. 2002;4(4):226-36.

18. Wampold BE. *The Great Psychotherapy Debate: Models, Methods, and Findings*. Mahwah, NJ: Lawrence Erlbaum Associates; 2001.

19. Bortolotti B, Menchetti M, Bellini F, Montaguti MB, Berardi D. Psychological interventions for major depression in primary care: a meta-analytic review of randomized controlled trials. Gen Hosp Psychiatry. 2008;30(4):293-302.

20. Butler AC, Chapman JE, Forman EM, Beck AT. The empirical status of cognitive-behavioral therapy: a review of meta-analyses. Clin Psychol Rev. 2006;26(1):17-31.

21. Craighead WE, Sheets ES, Brosse AL, Ilardi SS. Psychosocial treatments for major depressive disorder. In: Nathan PE, Gorman JM, eds. *A guide to treatments that work*. 3rd ed. New York: Oxford; 2007:289-293.

22. DeRubeis RJ, Gelfand LA, Tang TZ, Simons AD. Medications versus cognitive behavior therapy for severely depressed outpatients: mega-analysis of four randomized comparisons. Am J Psychiatry. 1999;156(7):1007-13.

23. DeRubeis RJ, Hollon SD, Amsterdam JD, et al. Cognitive therapy vs medications in the treatment of moderate to severe depression. Archives of General Psychiatry. 2005;62(4):409-16.

24. Pampallona S, Bollini P, Tibaldi G, Kupelnick B, Munizza C. Combined pharmacotherapy and psychological treatment for depression: a systematic review. Archives of General Psychiatry. 2004;61(7):714-9.

25. de Maat SM, Dekker J, Schoevers RA, de Jonghe F. Relative efficacy of psychotherapy and combined therapy in the treatment of depression: a meta-analysis. Eur Psychiatry. 2007;22(1):1-8.

26. Fava M, Rush AJ. Current status of augmentation and combination treatments for major depressive disorder: a literature review and a proposal for a novel approach to improve practice. Psychother Psychosom. 2006;75(3):139-53.

27. Segal Z, Vincent P, Levitt A. Efficacy of combined, sequential and crossover psychotherapy and pharmacotherapy in improving outcomes in depression. J Psychiatry Neurosci. 2002;27(4):281-90.

28. Cornwall PL, Scott J. Partial remission in depressive disorders. Acta Psychiatr Scand. 1997;95(4):265-71.

29. Fava M. Diagnosis and definition of treatment-resistant depression. Biol Psychiatry. 2003;53(8):649-59.

30. Stimpson N, Agrawal N, Lewis G. Randomised controlled trials investigating pharmacological and psychological interventions for treatment-refractory depression. Systematic review. Br J Psychiatry. 2002;181:284-94.

31. Trivedi MH. Major depressive disorder: remission of associated symptoms. J Clin Psychiatry. 2006;67 Suppl 6:27-32.

32. Rush AJ, Fava M, Wisniewski SR, et al. Sequenced treatment alternatives to relieve depression (STAR*D): rationale and design. Controlled Clinical Trials. 2004;25(1):119-42.

33. Rush AJ, Wisniewski SR, Warden D, et al. Selecting among second-step antidepressant medication monotherapies: predictive value of clinical, demographic, or first-step treatment features. Archives of General Psychiatry. 2008;65(8):870-80.

34. Corey-Lisle PK, Nash R, Stang P, Swindle R. Response, Partial Response, and Nonresponse in Primary Care Treatment of Depression. Archives of Internal Medicine. 2004;164(11):1197-1204.

35. Sherbourne C, Schoenbaum M, Wells KB, Croghan TW. Characteristics, treatment patterns, and outcomes of persistent depression despite treatment in primary care. General Hospital Psychiatry. 2004;26(2):106-14.

36. Souery D, Oswald P, Massat I, et al. Clinical factors associated with treatment resistance in major depressive disorder: results from a European multicenter study. Journal of Clinical Psychiatry. 2007;68(7):1062-70.

37. Thase ME, Friedman ES, Biggs MM, et al. Cognitive therapy versus medication in augmentation and switch strategies as second-step treatments: a STAR*D report. American Journal of Psychiatry. 2007;164(5):739-52.

38. Markowitz JC. When should psychotherapy be the treatment of choice for major depressive disorder? Current Psychiatry Reports. 2008;10(6):452-7.

39. Mitchell AJ. Depressed patients and treatment adherence. Lancet. 2006;367(9528):2041-3.

40.   Scott J, Teasdale JD, Paykel ES, et al. Effects of cognitive therapy on psychological symptoms and social functioning in residual depression. British Journal of Psychiatry. 2000;177:440-6.

41.   Harley R, Sprich S, Safren S, Jacobo M, Fava M. Adaptation of dialectical behavior therapy skills training group for treatment-resistant depression. Journal of Nervous and Mental Disease. 2008;196(2):136-43.

42.   Kennedy SH, Segal ZV, Cohen NL, Levitan RD, Gemar M, Bagby RM. Lithium carbonate versus cognitive therapy as sequential combination treatment strategies in partial responders to antidepressant medication: an exploratory trial. Journal of Clinical Psychiatry. 2003;64(4):439-44.

43.   Paykel ES, Scott J, Cornwall PL, et al. Duration of relapse prevention after cognitive therapy in residual depression: follow-up of controlled trial. Psychological Medicine. 2005;35(1):59-68.

44.   Paykel ES, Scott J, Teasdale JD, et al. Prevention of relapse in residual depression by cognitive therapy: a controlled trial. Archives of General Psychiatry. 1999;56(9):829-35.

45.   Scott J, Palmer S, Paykel E, Teasdale J, Hayhurst H. Use of cognitive therapy for relapse prevention in chronic depression. Cost-effectiveness study. British Journal of Psychiatry. 2003;182:221-7.

46.   Teasdale JD, Scott J, Moore RG, Hayhurst H, Pope M, Paykel ES. How does cognitive therapy prevent relapse in residual depression? Evidence from a controlled trial. Journal of Consulting and Clinical Psychology. 2001;69(3):347-57.

47.   Rush AJ, Trivedi MH, Wisniewski SR, et al. Acute and longer-term outcomes in depressed outpatients requiring one or several treatment steps: a STAR*D report. American Journal of Psychiatry. 2006;163(11):1905-17.

48.   Wisniewski SR, Fava M, Trivedi MH, et al. Acceptability of second-step treatments to depressed outpatients: a STAR*D report. American Journal of Psychiatry. 2007;164(5):753-60.

49.   Blackburn IM, Moore RG. Controlled acute and follow-up trial of cognitive therapy and pharmacotherapy in out-patients with recurrent depression. British Journal of Psychiatry. 1997;171:328-34.

50.   Wolf NJ, Hopko DR. Psychosocial and pharmacological interventions for depressed adults in primary care: a critical review. Clinical Psychology Review. 2008;28(1):131-61.

51.   Bower P, Gilbody S, Richards D, Fletcher J, Sutton A. Collaborative care for depression in primary care. Making sense of a complex intervention: systematic review and meta-regression. Br J Psychiatry. 2006;189:484-93.

52.   Lave JR, Frank RG, Schulberg HC, Kamlet MS. Cost-effectiveness of treatments for major depression in primary care practice. Archives of General Psychiatry. 1998;55(7):645-51.

53.   Barrett B, Byford S, Knapp M. Evidence of cost-effective treatments for depression: a systematic review. J Affect Disord. 2005;84(1):1-13.

54.   Leff J, Vearnals S, Brewin CR, et al. The London Depression Intervention Trial. Randomised controlled trial of antidepressants v. couple therapy in the treatment and maintenance of people with depression living with a partner: clinical outcome and costs. British Journal of Psychiatry. 2000;177:95-100.

55.   Simpson S, Corney R, Fitzgerald P, Beecham J. A randomized controlled trial to evaluate the effectiveness and cost-effectiveness of psychodynamic counselling for general practice patients with chronic depression. Psychological Medicine. 2003;33(2):229-39.

56.   Mynors-Wallis L, Davies I, Gray A, Barbour F, Gath D. A randomised controlled trial and cost analysis of problem-solving treatment for emotional disorders given by community nurses in primary care. Br J Psychiatry. 1997;170:113-9.

57.   Guthrie E, Moorey J, Margison F, et al. Cost-effectiveness of brief psychodynamic-interpersonal therapy in high utilizers of psychiatric services. Arch Gen Psychiatry. 1999;56(6):519-26.

58.   Russell JM, Hawkins K, Ozminkowski RJ, et al. The cost consequences of treatment-resistant depression. J Clin Psychiatry. 2004;65(3):341-7.

59.   Unutzer J, Katon W, Callahan CM, et al. Collaborative care management of late-life depression in the primary care setting: a randomized controlled trial. JAMA. 2002;288(22):2836-45.

60.   Williams JW, Jr., Gerrity M, Holsinger T, Dobscha S, Gaynes B, Dietrich A. Systematic review of multifaceted interventions to improve depression care. Gen Hosp Psychiatry. 2007;29(2):91-116.

61.   Katon W, Von Korff M, Lin E, et al. Stepped collaborative care for primary care patients with persistent symptoms of depression: a randomized trial. Arch Gen Psychiatry. 1999;56(12):1109-15.

62.   Williams JM, Teasdale JD, Segal ZV, Soulsby J. Mindfulness-based cognitive therapy reduces overgeneral autobiographical memory in formerly depressed patients. Journal of Abnormal Psychology. 2000;109(1):150-5.

63.   Bruce ML, Ten Have TR, Reynolds CF, 3rd, et al. Reducing suicidal ideation and depressive symptoms in depressed older primary care patients: a randomized controlled trial. JAMA. 2004;291(9):1081-91.

www.ingramcontent.com/pod-product-compliance
Lightning Source LLC
Chambersburg PA
CBHW081405170526
45166CB00010B/3213